SOUTH BEACH DIET COOKBOOK 2023

Quick and Easy Recipes in 30 Minutes to Lose Weight Fast and Have a Better Health, Plus Delicious and Friendly Recipes

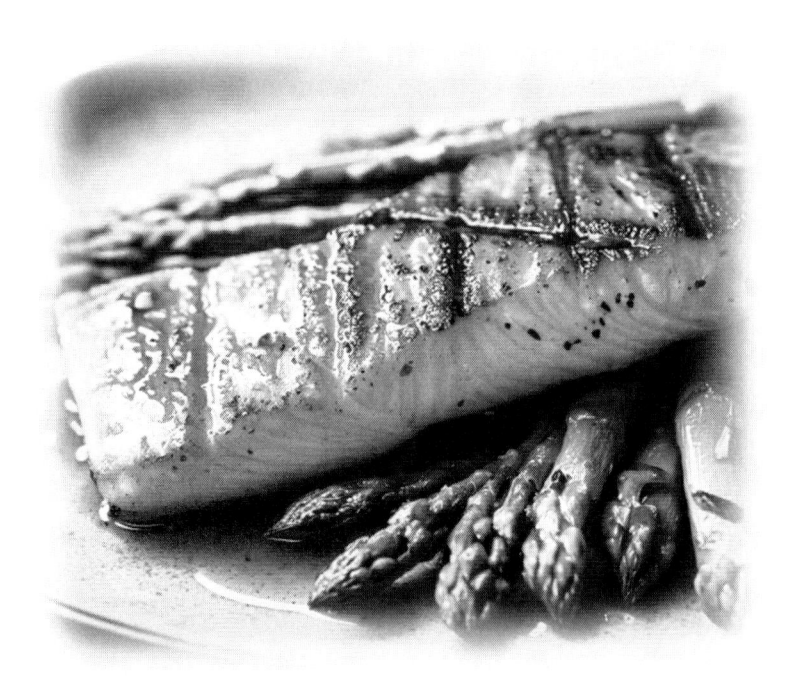

Kristy Nolan

Copyright©2023 Kristy Nolan

All Rights Reserved

No portion of this book may be reproduced in any form without permission from the publisher, except as permitted by U.S. copyright law.

INTRODUCTION 5

HOW TO USE THIS COOKBOOK 7

THE BENEFITS OF QUICK AND EASY RECIPES: 11

CHAPTER 1 17

   BREAKFASTS 17
      High-Protein Omelet with Spinach and Feta 17
      Greek Yogurt Parfait with Berries and Almonds 19
      Avocado and Egg Toast 20
      Turkey Bacon, and Veggie Frittata 21
      Chocolate Almond Smoothie 23
      Grilled Shrimp and Vegetable Skewers 23

CHAPTER 2 27

   SNACKS AND APPETIZERS 27
      Spicy Roasted Chickpeas 27
      Baked Zucchini Chips 29
      Deviled Eggs with Smoked Salmon 30
      Cucumber and Cream Cheese Roll-Ups 32
      Here are two additional recipes to add to Snacks and Appetizers with their instructions, ingredients, and benefits ... 34
      Mediterranean Chickpea Salad 34
      Mini Caprese Skewers 36

CHAPTER 3 39

   SOUPS AND SALADS 39
      Creamy Cauliflower Soup 39

- Chicken and Vegetable Soup 41
- Cobb Salad with Grilled Chicken 42
- Arugula and Quinoa Salad with Lemon Vinaigrette 44
- Here are two bonus recipes and their benefits 46
- Tomato and Basil Salad 46
- Lentil Soup 47

CHAPTER 4 50

MAIN COURSES 51
- Grilled Salmon with Asparagus 51
- Lemon-Garlic Chicken Thighs 53
- Balsamic-Glazed Pork Tenderloin 54
- Cauliflower Fried Rice with Shrimp 56

CHAPTER 5 61

SIDE DISHES 61
- Garlic and Herb Roasted Brussels Sprouts 61
- Sauteed Kale with Garlic and Lemon 63
- Broiled Asparagus with Parmesan 64
- Here's a bonus recipe and its benefits: 67
- Roasted Root Vegetables 67

CHAPTER 6 71

DESSERTS 71
- Chocolate Avocado Pudding 71
- Berry and Yogurt Parfait 73
- Peanut Butter and Banana Bites 74

- Greek Yogurt with Honey and Walnuts 76
- Here are two more bonus recipes for this chapter, along with their benefits: 76
- Dark Chocolate Bark with Nuts and Berries 77
- Baked Apple Chips 78

CHAPTER 7 81

- EXERCISE AND THE SOUTH BEACH DIET 81
  - Recommended Exercise Routines 83
  - Tips for Incorporating Exercise into Your Lifestyle 84

CHAPTER 8 88

- FREQUENTLY ASKED QUESTIONS ABOUT THE SOUTH BEACH DIET 88

CHAPTER 9 94

- TIPS FOR LONG-TERM SUCCESS WITH THE DIET 94

CONCLUSION 98

INTRODUCTION

Welcome to the South Beach Diet Express Cookbook! This cookbook is a collection of quick and easy recipes designed to help you achieve your health and weight loss goals. The South Beach Diet is a popular eating plan that emphasizes nutrient-dense foods, lean proteins, and healthy fats while avoiding processed foods and sugars.

The South Beach Diet is a proven weight loss program that has helped millions of people around the world achieve their health and fitness goals. This cookbook focuses on the "Express" version of the South Beach Diet, which is designed for people who have busy schedules and want to eat healthy, delicious meals without spending hours in the kitchen.

The recipes in this cookbook are designed to be easy to prepare, with most of them taking less than 30 minutes to make. Each recipe is crafted to include lean proteins, non-starchy vegetables, and healthy fats, which are the foundation of the South Beach Diet. You'll find recipes for breakfast, lunch, dinner, and snacks, as well as tips and tricks for making healthy eating a sustainable part of your lifestyle.

We hope that this cookbook will be a valuable resource for you on your journey to a healthier, happier you. With its tasty and easy-to-prepare recipes, you'll be able to enjoy nutritious and delicious meals without sacrificing flavor or convenience. Let's get started!

How to Use This Cookbook

The South Beach Diet Express Cookbook is designed to make healthy eating easy, convenient, and enjoyable. To get the most out of this cookbook, we suggest that you read through the following tips and guidelines before diving into the recipes:

Familiarize Yourself with the South Beach Diet: Before you begin using this cookbook, it's important to understand the principles of the South Beach Diet. This eating plan emphasizes lean proteins, non-starchy vegetables, and healthy fats while avoiding refined carbohydrates and sugars. By following the South Beach Diet, you'll not only lose weight, but you'll also improve your overall health and well-being.

Make a Meal Plan:

Planning your meals ahead of time can help you stay on track with your weight loss and health goals. This cookbook includes over 75 quick and easy recipes that are perfect for busy people who want to eat healthy without spending hours in the kitchen. Take some time to plan your meals for the week and choose the recipes that you want to make.

Stock Up on Staples:

Many of the recipes in this cookbook call for basic ingredients like olive oil, salt, and pepper. Make sure that you have these staples on hand, so that you can whip up a healthy meal whenever you need to. You may also want to stock up on non-perishable items like canned tomatoes and beans, which can be used in a variety of recipes.

Get Creative with Substitutions:

If you don't have all of the ingredients that a recipe calls for, don't worry! You can often substitute one ingredient for another without compromising the flavor or nutrition of the recipe. For example, you can substitute chicken for turkey or tofu for beef. Don't be afraid to experiment and get creative with your substitutions.

Double the Recipe:

Many of the recipes in this cookbook can be doubled or tripled, which is great for meal prep or feeding a larger family. If you have leftovers, you can store them in the refrigerator or freezer and enjoy them later.

Have Fun and Enjoy the Process:

Cooking should be enjoyable, not stressful! Take your time, experiment with flavors and ingredients, and don't be afraid to make mistakes. Remember, cooking is a learning process, and every mistake is an opportunity to improve your skills.

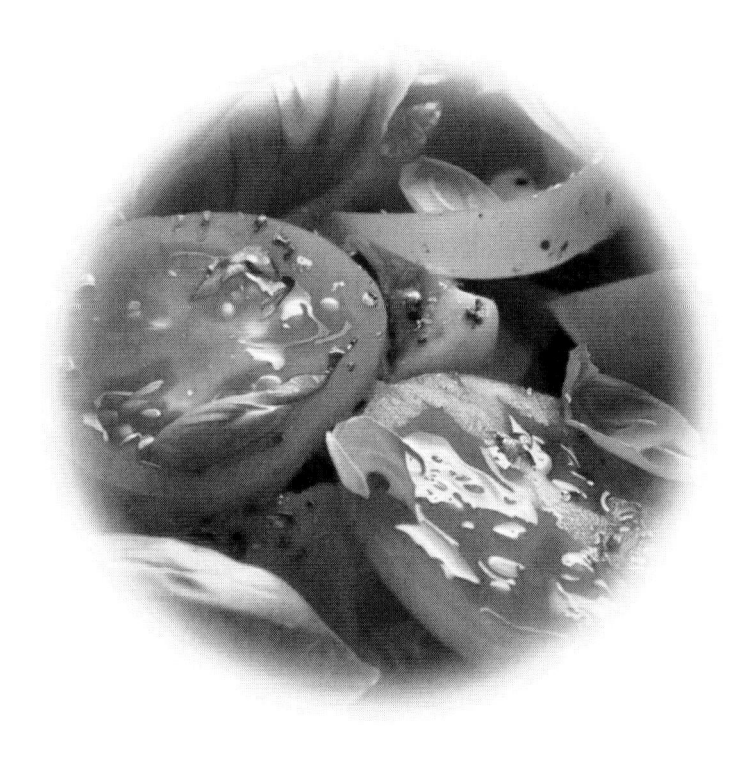

The Benefits of Quick and Easy Recipes:

The recipes in this cookbook are designed to be quick and easy, which means that you can spend less time in the kitchen and more time doing the things that you love. Here are some of the benefits of quick and easy recipes:

Save Time:

One of the biggest benefits of quick and easy recipes is that they save you time. By using simple ingredients and cooking techniques, you can prepare healthy meals in a fraction of the time that it would take to make more complex recipes.

Increase Convenience:

Quick and easy recipes are also convenient, especially for busy people who don't have a lot of time to spend in the kitchen. These recipes are perfect for weeknight dinners, lunch prep, and even breakfast on-the-go.

Promote Weight Loss:

Many of the recipes in this cookbook are designed to promote weight loss by incorporating lean proteins, non-starchy vegetables, and healthy fats. By following the South Beach Diet and cooking with these ingredients, you can achieve your weight loss goals and improve your overall health.

Improve Nutrition:

Quick and easy recipes can also help you improve your nutrition by using fresh, whole ingredients. By avoiding processed foods and sugars, you'll be able to fuel your body with the nutrients that it needs to function at its best.

Increase Confidence in the Kitchen:

Cooking can be intimidating. By mastering simple and efficient cooking techniques, you'll not only be able to whip up healthy and delicious meals in no time, but you'll also gain confidence in your ability to cook. This newfound confidence can be incredibly empowering, especially if you're someone who has always felt intimidated by the kitchen.

As you become more comfortable in the kitchen, you may even find that you start to experiment with different ingredients and techniques, branching out from the recipes in this cookbook to create your own signature dishes. And the more you cook, the more you'll learn about how different flavors and ingredients work together, allowing you to create even more delicious and nutritious meals in the future.

Another benefit of quick and easy recipes is that they often require minimal ingredients, making it easier to shop for and prepare meals. With fewer ingredients to work with, you can focus on quality rather than quantity, choosing the freshest and healthiest options available. Plus, you won't have to spend as much time and money at the grocery store, and you'll be less likely to waste food.

In addition to being convenient and efficient, quick and easy recipes can also be incredibly nutritious. The South Beach Diet emphasizes lean proteins and healthy fats, which are essential for supporting weight loss and maintaining overall health. By incorporating these foods into your diet in creative and delicious ways, you can ensure that you're getting the nutrients your body needs to thrive.

Of course, one of the biggest benefits of quick and easy recipes is that they allow you to save time without sacrificing flavor. With this cookbook, you'll discover a wide range of mouthwatering recipes that can be prepared in 30 minutes or less, from hearty breakfasts and satisfying lunches to indulgent dinners and sweet treats. Whether you're a busy professional, a parent on the go, or simply looking for delicious and healthy meals that won't take up too much of your time, this cookbook has something for everyone.

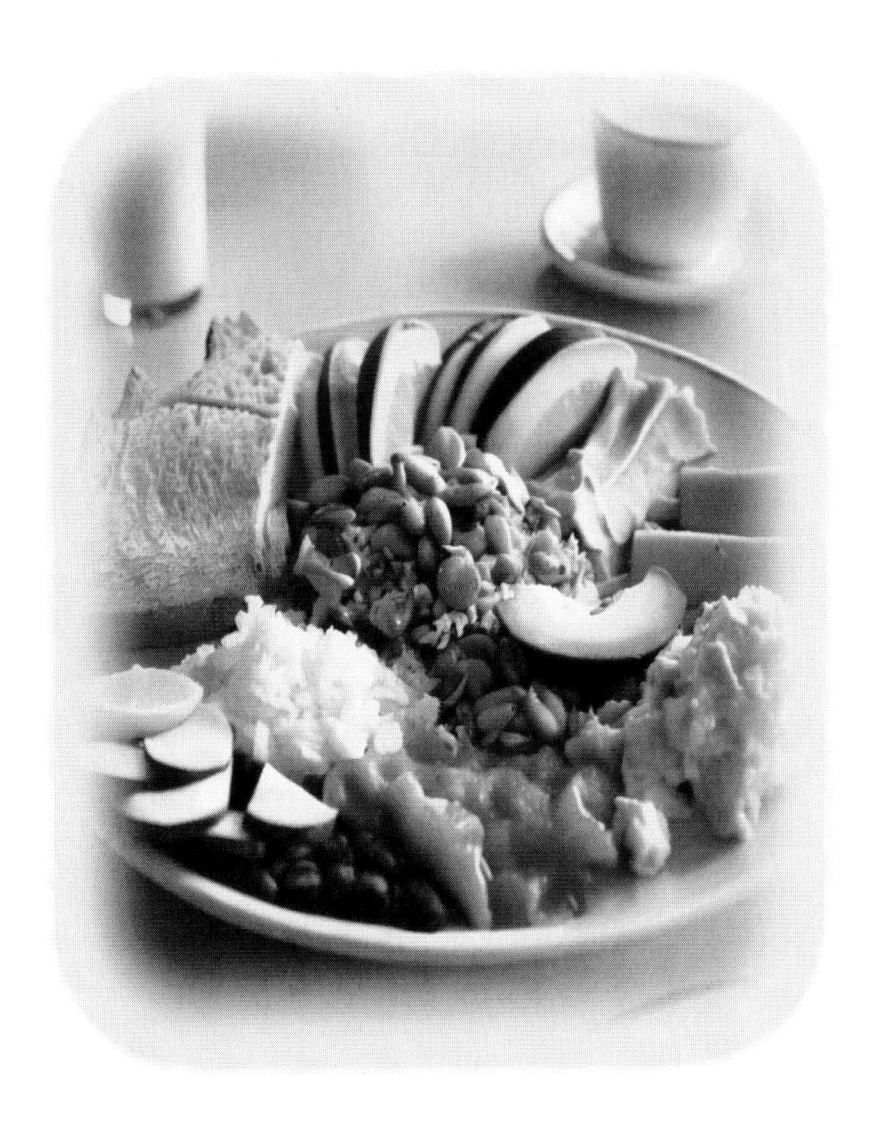

Chapter 1

Breakfasts

Starting your day off right is essential to achieving success on the South Beach Diet. Chapter 1 focuses on breakfasts that are not only quick and easy to make but also high in protein to keep you feeling full and satisfied throughout the morning.

High-Protein Omelet with Spinach and Feta

Ingredients:

2 large eggs

1/4 cup crumbled feta cheese

1/4 cup fresh spinach leaves, chopped

1/4 teaspoon salt

1/4 teaspoon black pepper

1 teaspoon olive oil

Instructions:

1. Put the eggs in a small bowl and proceed to beat them with a fork. Add the feta cheese, spinach, salt, and pepper and stir until well combined.
2. Heat the olive oil in a non-stick skillet over medium heat.
3. Pour the egg mixture into the skillet and cook for 2-3 minutes or until the bottom is set.
4. Use a spatula to fold the omelet in half and cook for an additional 1-2 minutes or until the eggs are cooked through.

Greek Yogurt Parfait with Berries and Almonds

Ingredients:

1 cup nonfat Greek yogurt

Half cup of mixed berries (like as strawberries, blueberries, and raspberries)

2 tablespoons sliced almonds

1/2 teaspoon honey

Instructions:

1. Put the Greek Yoghurt and honey in a small bowl and mix them thoroughly.
2. In a separate bowl, mix together the berries and almonds.
3. In a parfait glass or bowl, layer the yogurt mixture and the berry mixture, starting with the yogurt and ending with the berries.

Avocado and Egg Toast

Ingredients:

1 slice whole-grain bread, toasted

1/2 avocado, mashed

1 large egg, cooked to your liking

Salt and black pepper to taste

Instructions:

1. Toast the bread and spread the mashed avocado on top.
2. Cook the egg to your liking (scrambled, fried, or boiled) and place it on top of the avocado toast.
3. Sprinkle with salt and black pepper to taste.

Turkey Bacon, and Veggie Frittata

Ingredients:

6 large eggs
1/4 cup milk
1/2 cup diced turkey bacon
1/2 cup chopped mixed vegetables (such as bell peppers, onions, and mushrooms)
1/4 teaspoon salt
1/4 teaspoon black pepper
1 tablespoon olive oil

Instructions:

1. Preheat the oven to 375°F.
2. In a medium bowl, beat the eggs and milk with a fork. Add the turkey bacon, vegetables, salt, and pepper and stir until well combined.

3. In a safe for oven use pan over a medium-high flame, heat the olive oil.
4. Pour in the egg combo into the pan and cook for like 2-3 minutes or until the bottom is well cooked.
5. Transfer the skillet to the preheated oven and bake for 10-12 minutes or until the eggs are cooked through.

Enjoy these delicious and nutritious breakfast options to start your day off right on the South Beach Diet.

Here are two bonus recipes that would be great additions to your South Beach Diet Breakfast:

Chocolate Almond Smoothie

This delicious smoothie is a great breakfast or snack option that's packed with protein and healthy fats.

Simply blend together 1 cup unsweetened almond milk, 1 scoop chocolate protein powder, 1 tablespoon almond butter, 1/2 frozen banana, and 1/2 cup ice until smooth. Enjoy the rich, chocolatey flavor while also benefiting from the antioxidants found in cacao, the healthy fats in almond butter, and the potassium and fiber in banana.

Grilled Shrimp and Vegetable Skewers

These skewers are a perfect option for a quick and easy lunch or dinner that's also low-carb and high-protein.

Simply thread shrimp, cherry tomatoes, bell peppers, and zucchini onto skewers and brush with olive oil and seasonings of your choice. Grill for about 2-3 minutes per side until the shrimp is cooked through and the vegetables are slightly charred. Not only is this dish delicious, but it also provides a variety of essential vitamins and minerals found in the vegetables, and the protein in the shrimp helps to keep you full and satisfied.

The benefits of these recipes are clear. The Chocolate Almond Smoothie provides a nutritious and filling breakfast or snack option that is high in protein and healthy fats. The smoothie contains antioxidants, potassium, and fiber from the banana, which are essential nutrients that support overall health. The Grilled Shrimp and Vegetable Skewers offer a low-carb and high-protein meal that is easy to prepare and perfect for a quick lunch or dinner. The dish is packed with essential vitamins and minerals from the vegetables, and the protein in the shrimp helps to build and repair muscles while keeping you full for longer. These bonus recipes are a great addition to your South Beach Diet Express Cookbook and will provide your readers with even more delicious and healthy meal options.

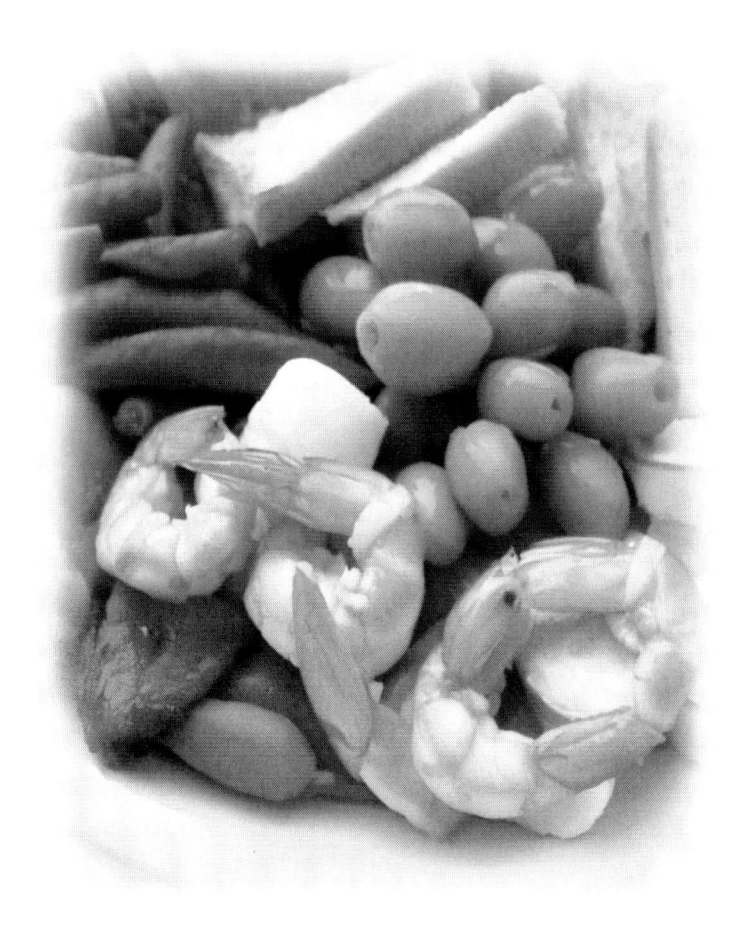

Chapter 2

Snacks and Appetizers

Snacks and appetizers are important components of any diet plan. They help to stave off hunger between meals, provide a quick energy boost, and can even help to control cravings. However, many snacks and appetizers are loaded with unhealthy fats, sugars, and other ingredients that can sabotage your weight loss goals. In this chapter, we'll explore some delicious and healthy snack and appetizer options that are perfect for the South Beach Diet.

Spicy Roasted Chickpeas

Chickpeas, also known as garbanzo beans, are a great source of protein and fiber, making them an excellent choice for a healthy snack. When roasted, they become crunchy and satisfying, and the addition of spices gives them an extra kick of flavor.

Ingredients:

1 can of chickpeas, drained and rinsed

1 tablespoon olive oil

1/2 teaspoon cumin

1/2 teaspoon chili powder

1/2 teaspoon paprika

Salt and pepper, to taste

Instructions:

1. Preheat the oven to 400°F (200°C).
2. In a bowl, combine the chickpeas, olive oil, cumin, chili powder, and paprika. Add salt and pepper to season it to your taste.
3. Spread the chickpeas out in a single layer on a baking sheet.

4. Bake for 20-25 minutes, stirring occasionally, until they are crispy and golden brown.
5. Let the chickpeas cool for a few minutes before serving.

Baked Zucchini Chips

Potato chips may be a tempting snack, but they are loaded with unhealthy fats and calories. Baked zucchini chips are a great alternative that are just as crunchy and satisfying, but much healthier.

Ingredients

2 medium zucchinis, sliced into thin rounds
1/2 cup almond flour
1/2 teaspoon garlic powder
1/2 teaspoon dried basil

1/2 teaspoon dried oregano

Salt and pepper, to taste

1 egg, beaten

Instructions:

1. Preheat the oven to 425°F (220°C).
2. In a bowl, combine the almond flour, garlic powder, dried basil, dried oregano, salt, and pepper.
3. Dip each zucchini slice in the beaten egg, then coat it in the almond flour mixture.
4. Place the coated zucchini slices in a single layer on a baking sheet.
5. Bake for 20-25 minutes, until the zucchini chips are crispy and golden brown.

Deviled Eggs with Smoked Salmon

Ingredients:

6 hard-boiled eggs, peeled

2 oz smoked salmon, chopped

2 tbsp mayonnaise

1 tbsp Dijon mustard

1 tbsp lemon juice

Salt and pepper, to taste

Dill, for garnish

Instructions:

1. Extract the yolks from the egg that has been hard-boiled by cutting them in half horizontally.
2. In a mixing bowl, combine the egg yolks, smoked salmon, mayonnaise, Dijon mustard, and lemon juice.
3. Mix everything together until smooth and creamy.
4. Add pepper and salt as it suits your taste.

5. Using a spoon, fill each egg white half with the yolk mixture.
6. Garnish each deviled egg with a sprig of fresh dill.
7. Serve chilled.

Benefits: Deviled eggs with smoked salmon are a great source of protein and healthy fats. The combination of the egg yolk and salmon provides a good amount of omega-3 fatty acids, which have been linked to many health benefits, including reducing inflammation and improving brain health.

Cucumber and Cream Cheese Roll-Ups

Ingredients:

1 large cucumber

4 oz cream cheese, softened

1 tbsp fresh dill, chopped

1 tbsp fresh parsley, chopped

Salt and pepper, to taste

Instructions:

1. Cut the cucumber lengthwise into thin slices using a mandoline or vegetable peeler.
2. In a mixing bowl, combine the cream cheese, dill, parsley, salt, and pepper.
3. Mix everything together until smooth and creamy.
4. Take a cucumber slice and spread a layer of the cream cheese mixture on top.
5. Roll up the cucumber slice, making sure the cream cheese mixture is evenly distributed.
6. Repeat with the remaining cucumber slices and cream cheese mixture.
7. Serve chilled.

Benefits: Cucumber and cream cheese roll-ups are a low-carb and low-calorie snack that is perfect for anyone following the South Beach Diet. Cucumbers are a good source of vitamins and minerals, while cream cheese provides a good amount of protein and healthy fats. The fresh herbs add a burst of flavor and provide additional health benefits, including reducing inflammation and improving digestion.

Here are two additional recipes to add to Snacks and Appetizers with their instructions, ingredients, and benefits.

Mediterranean Chickpea Salad
Ingredients:
1 can chickpeas, drained and rinsed
1/4 cup chopped red onion

1/4 cup chopped cucumber

1/4 cup chopped cherry tomatoes

1/4 cup crumbled feta cheese

2 tablespoons chopped fresh parsley

1 tablespoon extra-virgin olive oil

1 tablespoon lemon juice

Salt and black pepper to taste

Instructions:

1. In a mixing bowl, combine chickpeas, red onion, cucumber, cherry tomatoes, feta cheese, and parsley.
2. Drizzle with olive oil and lemon juice, and season with salt and black pepper to taste.
3. Toss well and serve.

Benefits: This Mediterranean chickpea salad is a great snack or appetizer option on the South Beach Diet. Chickpeas are strong in fiber as well as protein, so they keep you satisfied for more time and enable you to avoid cravings. The salad is also loaded with nutrient-dense vegetables like cucumber and tomatoes, which provide vitamins, minerals, and antioxidants. The feta cheese adds a tangy flavor and a dose of calcium, while the olive oil provides healthy fats that are good for your heart.

Mini Caprese Skewers

Ingredients:

12 cherry tomatoes

12 small fresh mozzarella balls

12 small basil leaves

1 tablespoon balsamic vinegar

1 tablespoon extra-virgin olive oil

Salt and black pepper to taste

Instructions:

1. Thread a cherry tomato, a mozzarella ball, and a basil leaf onto a small skewer.
2. Repeat with the remaining ingredients to make 12 skewers.
3. Drizzle with balsamic vinegar and olive oil, and season with salt and black pepper to taste.
4. Serve.

Benefits: These mini caprese skewers are a delicious and easy snack or appetizer that fits perfectly with the South Beach Diet. Cherry tomatoes are a good source of vitamin C and lycopene, a powerful antioxidant that helps protect against cancer and heart disease. Fresh mozzarella provides protein and calcium, while basil adds a fresh and aromatic flavor. The balsamic vinegar and olive oil dressing add healthy fats and antioxidants that benefit your heart and overall health.

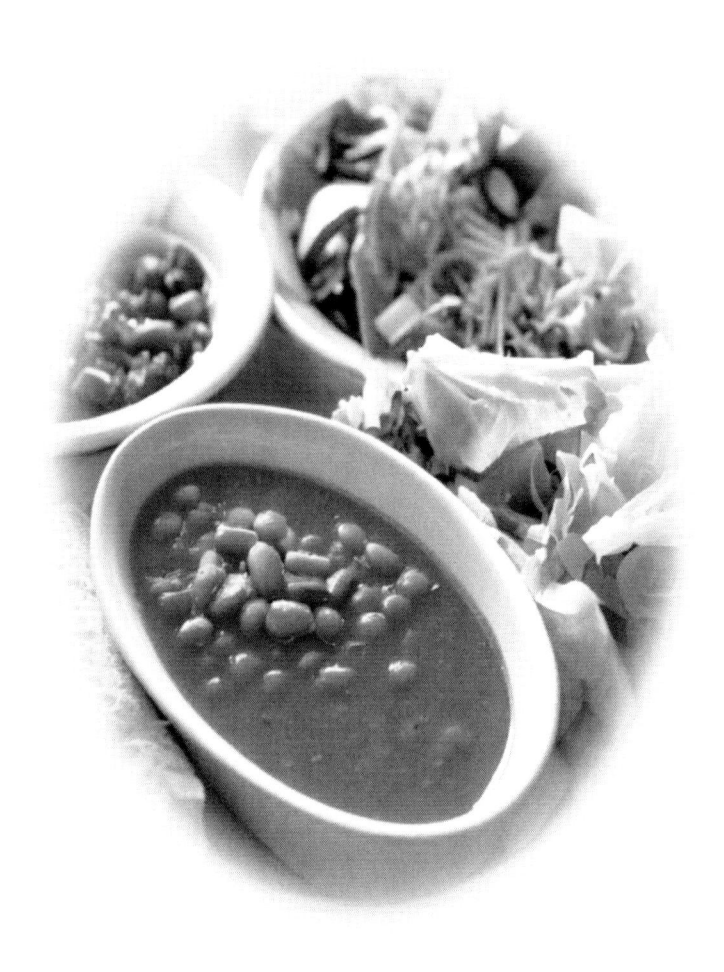

Chapter 3

Soups and Salads

Soups and salads can be a delicious and healthy addition to your South Beach Diet meal plan. Not only are they packed with essential nutrients, but they're also a great way to add variety to your diet. In this chapter, we'll share some of our favorite soup and salad recipes that are easy to make and perfect for any occasion.

Creamy Cauliflower Soup

This creamy cauliflower soup is a great way to get your daily dose of vegetables. It's rich and satisfying, and the addition of cream cheese makes it even more decadent. Here's what you'll need:

Ingredients:

1 head of cauliflower, chopped

1 onion, chopped

2 cloves of garlic, minced

4 cups of chicken broth

1/2 cup cream cheese

Salt and pepper to taste

Instructions

1. In a large pot, sauté the onion and garlic until fragrant.
2. Add the cauliflower and chicken broth, and bring to a boil.
3. Reduce the heat and simmer until the cauliflower is tender.
4. Remove from heat and let cool for a few minutes.

5. Using an immersion blender, blend the soup until smooth.
6. Add the cream cheese and stir until melted and well combined.
7. Season with salt and pepper to taste.

Chicken and Vegetable Soup

This chicken and vegetable soup is a hearty and satisfying meal that's perfect for any time of year. It's packed with protein and fiber, and the addition of vegetables makes it a healthy choice. Here's what you'll need:

Ingredients:

1 pound boneless, skinless chicken breasts, cubed

2 cups chopped mixed vegetables (carrots, celery, onions)

4 cups chicken broth

1/2 teaspoon dried thyme

Salt and pepper to taste

Instructions:

1. In a large pot, sauté the chicken until browned.
2. Add the chopped vegetables, chicken broth, and thyme.
3. Bring to a boil, then reduce heat and simmer until the vegetables are tender and the chicken is cooked through.
4. As it may please you, add salt and pepper to taste.

Cobb Salad with Grilled Chicken

Ingredients:

2 boneless, skinless chicken breasts

1 tsp. garlic powder

1 tsp. onion powder

Salt and black pepper, to taste

6 cups of mixed salad greens

4 slices of turkey bacon, cooked and crumbled

2 hard-boiled eggs, chopped

1 large tomato, chopped

1 avocado, chopped,

1/4 cup crumbled blue cheese

1/4 cup balsamic vinaigrette

Instructions:

1. Heat a grill or grill pan on medium-high. Season the chicken breasts with garlic powder, onion powder, salt, and pepper.
2. Grill the chicken for 6-7 minutes per side, or until cooked through.

3. Let the chicken rest for 5 minutes, then slice it into strips.
4. Separate the salad greens among four different plates and set aside.
5. Top each plate with turkey bacon, chopped eggs, tomato, avocado, and blue cheese.
6. Add the sliced chicken to each plate.
7. Drizzle with balsamic vinaigrette.

Arugula and Quinoa Salad with Lemon Vinaigrette

Ingredients:

1 cup cooked quinoa

4 cups of baby arugula

1/4 cup chopped fresh parsley

1/4 cup chopped fresh mint

1/4 cup chopped red onion

1/4 cup crumbled feta cheese

1/4 cup sliced almonds

1/4 cup olive oil

2 tbsp. lemon juice

1 tsp. honey

Salt and black pepper, to taste

Instructions:

1. In a large bowl, combine the cooked quinoa, arugula, parsley, mint, red onion, feta cheese, and almonds.
2. In a small bowl, whisk together the olive oil, lemon juice, honey, salt, and pepper.
3. Drizzle the dressing over the salad and toss to coat.
4. Serve immediately.

Here are two bonus recipes and their benefits

Tomato and Basil Salad

Ingredients:

4 medium tomatoes, sliced

1/2 cup fresh basil leaves, chopped

1/4 cup red onion, thinly sliced

2 tbsp. extra-virgin olive oil

1 tbsp balsamic vinegar

Salt and pepper, to taste

Instructions:

1. In a large bowl, combine the sliced tomatoes, chopped basil, and thinly sliced red onion.
2. Drizzle the extra-virgin olive oil and balsamic vinegar over the tomato mixture.

3. Season with salt and pepper to taste.
4. Toss everything together until well combined.
5. Serve and enjoy!

Benefits: This salad is rich in antioxidants, vitamins, and minerals, making it a great addition to a healthy diet. Tomatoes are high in lycopene, which has been linked to reducing the risk of cancer and heart disease. Basil is also rich in antioxidants and has anti-inflammatory properties, which can help improve digestion and reduce stress.

Lentil Soup

Ingredients:

1 cup dried lentils

1 onion, chopped

2 garlic cloves, minced

2 carrots, chopped

2 celery stalks, chopped

1 tbsp extra-virgin olive oil

4 cups chicken or vegetable broth

1 tsp dried thyme

1 bay leaf

Salt and pepper, to taste

Instructions:

1. Rinse the lentils in a colander and remove any debris or stones.
2. In a large pot or Dutch oven, heat the extra-virgin olive oil over medium heat.
3. Add the chopped onion, minced garlic, chopped carrots, and chopped celery to the pot. Sauté until the vegetables are tender and fragrant, about 5 minutes.

4. Add the rinsed lentils, chicken or vegetable broth, dried thyme, and bay leaf to the pot.
5. Bring the mixture to a boil, then reduce the heat and simmer for about 30 minutes, or until the lentils are tender.
6. Season with salt and pepper to taste.
7. Remove the bay leaf and serve hot.

Benefits: Lentils are a great source of plant-based protein and are high in fiber, making them a great food for weight loss and digestive health. They also contain folate, iron, and other important vitamins and minerals. This soup is also a great option for vegetarians and vegans, and it can be easily customized with different spices and vegetables.

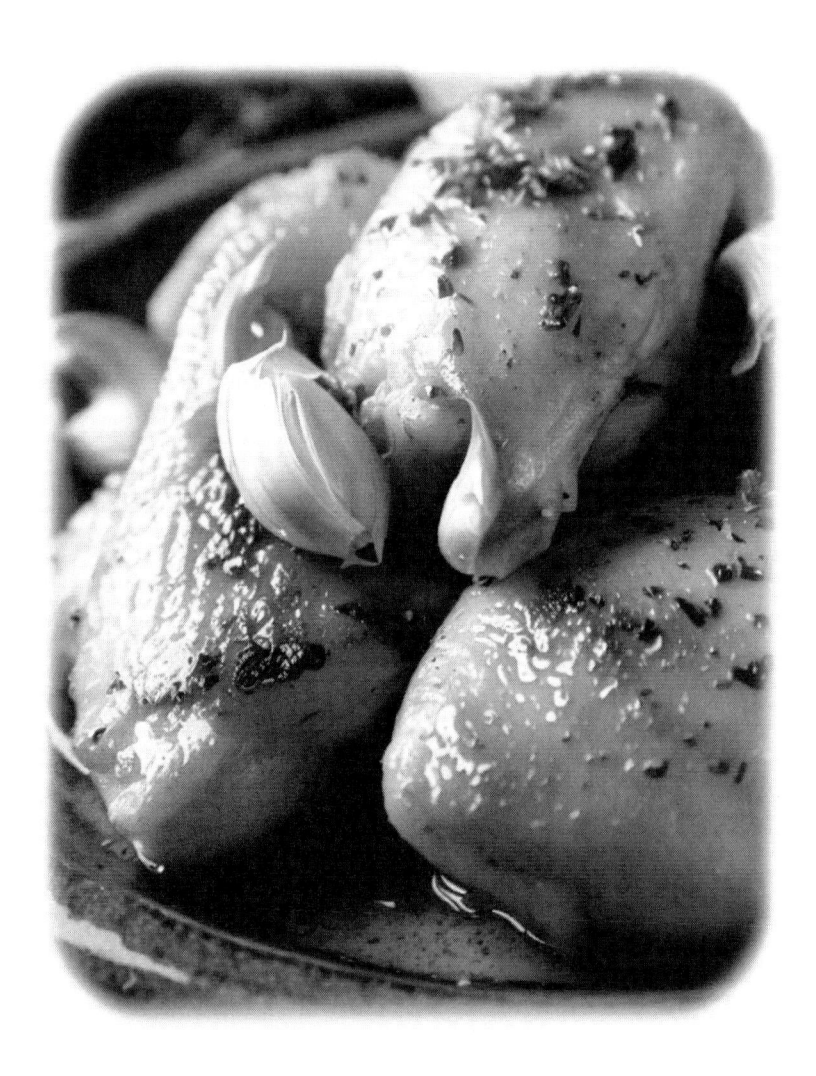

Chapter 4

Main Courses

This chapter is all about satisfying and healthy main courses that are perfect for any meal of the day. Whether you're cooking for yourself or a group of people, these dishes will surely impress.

Grilled Salmon with Asparagus

This grilled salmon with asparagus dish is a perfect meal for a healthy diet. Salmon is an excellent source of protein and omega-3 fatty acids that can help to reduce inflammation and promote heart health. Asparagus, on the other hand, is packed with fiber, vitamins, and minerals that are essential for good health.

Ingredients:

4 salmon filets

1 pound of asparagus

1 tablespoon olive oil

1/2 teaspoon salt

1/4 teaspoon black pepper

1/2 lemon

Instructions:

1. Preheat your grill to medium-high heat.
2. Toss the asparagus in olive oil and season with salt and black pepper.
3. Place the salmon filets and asparagus on the grill and cook for 4-5 minutes per side.
4. Squeeze fresh lemon juice over the salmon and serve.

Lemon-Garlic Chicken Thighs

This lemon-garlic chicken thigh recipe is a flavorful and easy-to-make dish that is perfect for a busy weeknight dinner. Chicken thighs are a great source of lean protein and iron, and the lemon and garlic add a burst of flavor to this dish.

Ingredients:

4 chicken thighs

1 lemon

4 garlic cloves

2 tablespoons of olive oil

1 teaspoon dried oregano

1/2 teaspoon salt

1/4 teaspoon black pepper

Instructions:

1. Preheat your oven to 375°F.

2. In a small bowl, whisk together the olive oil, minced garlic, oregano, salt, and black pepper.
3. Place the chicken thighs in a baking dish and pour the olive oil mixture over them, making sure to coat them well.
4. Cut the lemon into slices and place them on top of the chicken thighs.
5. Bake for 30-35 minutes, until the chicken is cooked through.

Balsamic-Glazed Pork Tenderloin

Ingredients:

1 pork tenderloin

1/4 cup balsamic vinegar

2 tbsp. honey

2 tbsp Dijon mustard

2 cloves of garlic, minced

1/4 tsp black pepper

Salt, to taste

1 tbsp olive oil

Instructions:

1. Preheat oven to 400°F.
2. In a small bowl, whisk together balsamic vinegar, honey, Dijon mustard, garlic, black pepper, and salt.
3. Take olive oil and heat it in a pan at a low flame.
4. Sear the pork tenderloin on all sides, about 2-3 minutes per side.
5. Brush the balsamic mixture onto the pork tenderloin.
6. Transfer the skillet to the preheated oven and bake for 20-25 minutes, or until the internal temperature of the pork reaches 145°F.

7. Remove the pork from the oven and let it rest for 5 minutes before slicing.

Benefits: Pork tenderloin is a lean protein that is rich in vitamins and minerals such as iron, zinc, and vitamin B12. Balsamic vinegar provides a tangy flavor and may offer potential health benefits, such as reducing blood sugar levels and improving digestion. This dish when prepared is gluten-free and low-carb.

Cauliflower Fried Rice with Shrimp

Ingredients:
1 head of cauliflower, grated into rice-sized pieces
1 lb. shrimp, peeled and deveined
2 cloves of garlic, minced
1 small onion, chopped

1 cup mixed frozen vegetables (such as peas, carrots, and corn)

3 tbsp. low-sodium soy sauce

2 tbsp sesame oil

2 eggs, beaten

Salt and black pepper, to taste

Green onions, sliced, for garnish

Instructions:

1. In a large skillet, heat 1 tbsp sesame oil over medium-high heat.
2. Add the shrimp and cook until pink and cooked through, about 2-3 minutes per side. Remove from skillet and set aside.
3. In the same skillet, add the remaining sesame oil and sauté garlic and onion until softened, about 3-4 minutes.

4. Add the grated cauliflower and frozen vegetables to the skillet and cook until tender, about 5-6 minutes.
5. Push the cauliflower mixture to the sides of the skillet and pour in the beaten eggs. Scramble the eggs until cooked through, then mix into the cauliflower mixture.
6. Add the cooked shrimp to the skillet and stir to combine.
7. Season with soy sauce, salt, and black pepper to taste. Slice some green onions and garnish it with them before serving.

Benefits: This dish is a healthier alternative to traditional fried rice, as it is lower in carbohydrates and higher in fiber. Cauliflower is a cruciferous vegetable that is packed with nutrients, including vitamin C, vitamin K, and folate. Shrimp is a low-fat source of protein that is also rich in omega-3 fatty acids, which may help reduce inflammation and improve heart health. This dish is also gluten-free and can be easily customized with your favorite vegetables and seasonings.

Overall, the recipes in this chapter offer a variety of options for main courses that are quick and easy to prepare, yet still satisfying and nutritious.

Chapter 5

Side Dishes

When it comes to meal planning, it's easy to focus on the main dish and forget about the sides. But side dishes are just as important as the main course, providing valuable nutrients and adding flavor and texture to your meal. In this chapter, we'll share some simple yet delicious side dish recipes that are easy to make and packed with nutrition.

Garlic and Herb Roasted Brussels Sprouts

Ingredients:

1 pound Brussels sprouts, trimmed and halved

2 tablespoons olive oil

2 cloves garlic, minced

1 teaspoon dried thyme

Salt and pepper to taste

Instructions:

1. Preheat the oven to 400°F.
2. In a large bowl, toss Brussels sprouts with olive oil, garlic, thyme, salt, and pepper.
3. On a sheet of baking parchment, arrange Brussels sprouts in just one layer.
4. Roast for 20-25 minutes, or until tender and lightly browned.

Benefits: Brussels sprouts are a great source of vitamin C, vitamin K, and fiber. Roasting them with garlic and herbs gives them a delicious flavor and makes them a perfect side dish for any meal.

Sauteed Kale with Garlic and Lemon

Ingredients:

A single bunch of kale, leaves and stems plucked

2 tablespoons olive oil

2 cloves garlic, minced

Juice of 1 lemon

Salt and pepper to taste

Instructions:

1. In a massive pan over a medium-high temperature, heat the olive oil.
2. Add garlic and cook for 1-2 minutes, or until fragrant.
3. Add kale and cook for 3-4 minutes, or until wilted.
4. Add lemon juice, salt, and pepper and stir to combine.

Benefits: Kale is one of the most nutrient-dense foods on the planet, packed with vitamins A, C, and K, as well as fiber and antioxidants. Sautéing it with garlic and lemon makes it a tasty and nutritious side dish that pairs well with any main course.

Broiled Asparagus with Parmesan

Ingredients:

1 pound asparagus, trimmed

2 tablespoons olive oil

1/4 cup grated Parmesan cheese

Salt and pepper to taste

Instructions:

1. Preheat the broiler.
2. Mix asparagus alongside olive oil, salt, and pepper to taste.

3. On a sheet of baking parchment, arrange the asparagus in just one layer.
4. Broil for 5-7 minutes, or until tender and lightly charred.
5. Sprinkle with Parmesan cheese and broil for an additional minute, or until cheese is melted and bubbly.

Benefits: Asparagus is a great source of vitamins A, C, and K, as well as folate and fiber. Broiling it with Parmesan cheese gives it a delicious flavor and makes it a perfect side dish for any meal.

Ingredients:

1 head of cauliflower, cut into florets
2 tbsp olive oil
1 tsp ground turmeric
1 tsp ground cumin
1/2 tsp salt

1/4 tsp black pepper

Instructions:
1. Preheat the oven to 400°F.
2. In a small bowl, mix together the olive oil, turmeric, cumin, salt, and black pepper.
3. Place the cauliflower florets on a baking sheet lined with parchment paper.
4. Drizzle the spice mixture over the cauliflower and toss to coat.
5. Roast in the oven for 20-25 minutes, or until the cauliflower is tender and lightly browned.
6. Serve immediately.

Benefits:

Cauliflower is a cruciferous vegetable that is packed with nutrients such as fiber, vitamin C, and folate. Turmeric and cumin are both spices that have anti-inflammatory properties, which can help reduce inflammation in the body. Roasting the cauliflower with these spices not only adds flavor but also increases the nutritional benefits of the dish.

Here's a bonus recipe and its benefits:

Roasted Root Vegetables

Ingredients:

2 cups cubed butternut squash

2 cups cubed sweet potato

2 cups cubed parsnip

2 cups cubed carrot

2 tbsp. olive oil

1 tsp. dried thyme

Salt and pepper, to taste

Instructions:

1. Preheat the oven to 425°F.

2. Place the cubed butternut squash, sweet potato, parsnip, and carrot in a large mixing bowl.
3. Drizzle olive oil over the vegetables and toss to coat evenly.
4. Sprinkle dried thyme, salt, and pepper over the vegetables and toss to coat evenly.
5. Transfer the vegetables to a baking sheet.
6. Roast in the oven for 25-30 minutes, or until the vegetables are fork-tender and golden brown.
7. Serve immediately.

Benefits of Roasted Root Vegetables

- Root vegetables are a great source of complex carbohydrates, fiber, and vitamins.
- Butternut squash is rich in beta-carotene, vitamin C, and potassium.

- Sweet potatoes are a good source of vitamin A, vitamin C, and fiber.
- Carrots are a great source of vitamin A, biotin, and potassium.
- Parsnips are a good source of fiber, vitamin C, and folate.
- Roasted root vegetables are a delicious and nutritious side dish that is easy to prepare and pairs well with a variety of main courses.

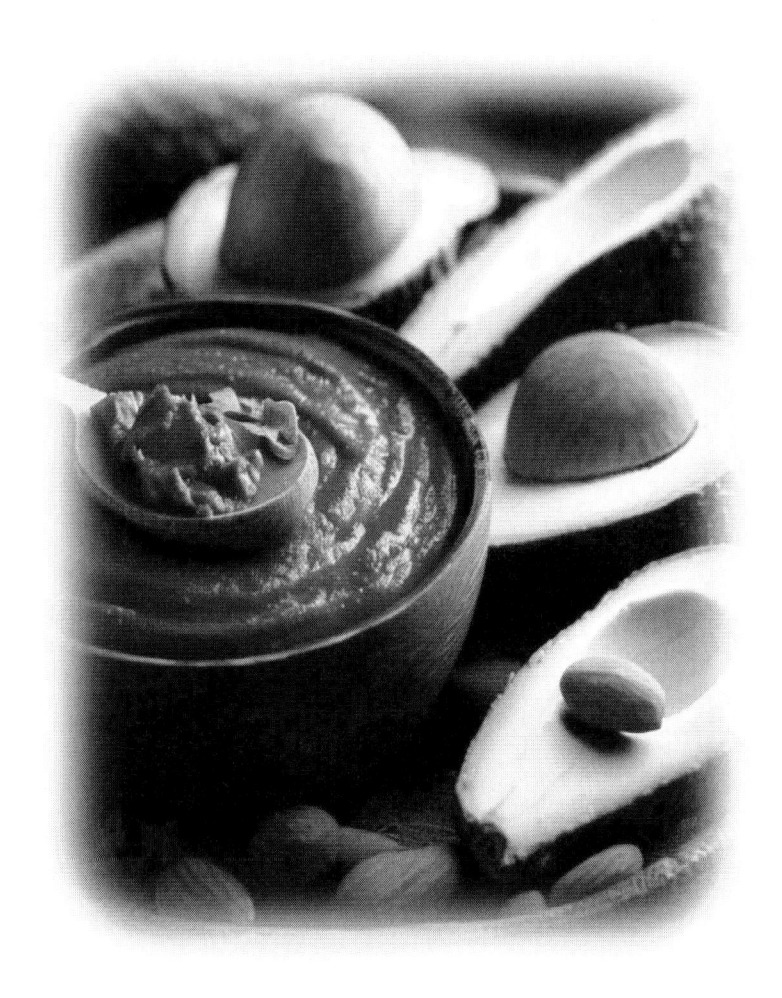

Chapter 6

Desserts

When it comes to healthy eating, it's important to remember that you don't have to give up all sweets and desserts. With the right ingredients and recipes, you can indulge your sweet tooth while still maintaining a healthy diet. In this chapter, we'll explore some delicious and nutritious dessert options that you can feel good about enjoying.

Chocolate Avocado Pudding

This creamy and decadent chocolate pudding is made with avocados, which are a great source of healthy fats, fiber, and potassium. It's also sweetened with maple syrup, which is a healthier alternative to refined sugar.

Ingredients:

This creamy and scrumptious chocolate pudding is made with avocados, which are abundant in healthy fats, fiber, and potassium. It's also sweetened with maple syrup, a healthier alternative to refined sugar.

Ingredients:

2 ripe avocados

1/2 cup unsweetened chocolate powder

1 tablespoon maple syrup

One-fourth cup almond milk

1 tsp vanilla extract 1 tsp salt

Instructions:

1. Remove the avocados' pits by halves them. Half-fill a blender or food processor with the flesh.

2. Combine the cocoa powder, maple syrup, almond milk, vanilla extract, and salt in a blender or food processor.
3. Scrape down the sides of the mixing bowl as needed until the mixture is smooth and creamy.
4. Refrigerate the pudding for at least 30 minutes before serving in a bowl or individual serving dishes.

Berry and Yogurt Parfait

Ingredients:

1 cup plain Greek yogurt

1 cup mixed berries (strawberries, blueberries, raspberries)

1/2 cup granola

1 tbsp honey

1 tsp vanilla extract

Instructions:

1. In a small bowl, mix together the Greek yogurt, honey, and vanilla extract.
2. The mixed berries should be combined in a different bowl.
3. In a parfait glass, layer the Greek yogurt mixture, granola, and mixed berries.
4. Layers should be repeated until the glass is filled.
5. Serve right away or keep chilled until you're ready to serve.

Peanut Butter and Banana Bites

Ingredients:

2 ripe bananas, sliced into rounds

1/4 cup natural peanut butter

1/4 cup dark chocolate chips

1 tbsp coconut oil

Instructions:

1. Lay the banana slices flat on a baking sheet lined with parchment paper.
2. In a small bowl, mix together the peanut butter and coconut oil.
3. Spoon a small amount of the peanut butter mixture onto each banana slice.
4. Sprinkle the dark chocolate chips on top of the peanut butter mixture.
5. Place the baking sheet in the freezer for 1-2 hours, or until the banana bites are frozen.
6. Remove from the freezer and serve immediately.

Greek Yogurt with Honey and Walnuts

Ingredients:

1 cup Greek yogurt, plain

2 tablespoons honey

1/4 cup walnuts, chopped

Instructions:

1. Combine the Greek yogurt and honey in a small mixing dish.
2. Top the yogurt mixture with the chopped walnuts.
3. Serve straight away or keep chilled until ready to use.

Here are two more bonus recipes for this chapter, along with their benefits:

Dark Chocolate Bark with Nuts and Berries

Ingredients:

8 oz. dark chocolate chips

1/2 cup mixed nuts (such as almonds, walnuts, and cashews)

1/2 cup mixed berries (such as blueberries, raspberries, and cranberries)

Instructions:

1. Heat the dark chips of chocolate in your microwave or a double boiler.
2. Line a baking sheet with parchment paper and spread the melted chocolate on top.
3. Sprinkle the mixed nuts and berries on top of the chocolate.
4. Place the baking sheet in the refrigerator for a period of between twenty-five to thirty 30

minutes, or until the chocolate must have hardened.
5. Break the chocolate bark into pieces and serve.

Benefits: Dark chocolate is high in antioxidants and can improve heart health. Nuts and berries are also rich in antioxidants and can help lower inflammation in the body.

Baked Apple Chips

Ingredients:

2 apples

1 tsp. cinnamon

1 tbsp. Honey

Instructions:

1. Preheat the oven to 200°F.
2. Slice the apples into thin rounds, removing the seeds and core.
3. In a small bowl, mix together the cinnamon and honey.
4. Dip each apple slice into the cinnamon-honey mixture, making sure both sides are coated.
5. Place the apple slices on a baking sheet lined with parchment paper.
6. Bake for 2-3 hours, or until the apple slices are crispy and lightly browned.
7. Allow to cool and store in a container that won't allow the entrance of air.

Benefits: Apples as a fruit are a great source of fiber and essential antioxidants. Cinnamon can help regulate blood sugar levels, and honey is a natural sweetener that can offer some health benefits over processed sugar.

CHAPTER 7

Exercise and the South Beach Diet

Exercise is an essential component of a healthy lifestyle, and it can be especially beneficial when combined with a healthy diet like the South Beach Diet. Exercise helps to burn calories, build lean muscle mass, and increase metabolism, all of which can help you achieve and maintain a healthy weight.

Here are some of the key benefits of exercise on the South Beach Diet:

Burns calories: Exercise is a great way to burn calories, which is essential for weight loss. When you burn more calories than you consume, your body will start to use stored fat for energy, which can help you shed excess pounds. By adding exercise to your South Beach Diet plan, you can speed up the weight loss process and achieve your goals more quickly.

Builds lean muscle mass: Exercise helps to build lean muscle mass, which is important for maintaining a healthy metabolism. The more muscle mass you have, the greater number of calories that your body will burn at rest since the tissue of muscles uses more calories than fat tissue. By incorporating strength training exercises into your workout routine, you can build lean muscle mass and increase your metabolism.

Increases metabolism: Exercise can increase your metabolism, which is the rate at which your body burns calories. You may burn more calories all day long, regardless of whether you're not exercising, by raising your metabolism. Long-term, this can assist you in achieving and maintaining a healthy weight.

Recommended Exercise Routines

When it comes to exercise, there are many different types of activities that you can do to support your South Beach Diet plan. Here are some recommended exercise routines:

Cardiovascular exercise: Exercise that raises the rate of your heart and breathing rate is referred to as cardiovascular exercise (or "cardio" for short). Cardiovascular exercises include vigorous walking, jogging, cycling, and swimming. Aim to do at least 30 minutes of cardio exercise each day to support your South Beach Diet plan.

Strength training: Strength training exercises help to build lean muscle mass and increase metabolism. Weightlifting, resistance band training, and bodyweight workouts like push-ups and squats are a few examples of strength training exercises. At least three to four times a week should be set aside for strength training.

Flexibility training: Flexibility training exercises, like yoga and stretching, can help improve your flexibility and range of motion, which can reduce your risk of injury and improve your overall fitness level. Aim to do flexibility training exercises at least two to three times per week.

Tips for Incorporating Exercise into Your Lifestyle

It can be difficult to know where to begin if you've never done any exercise before. Here are some pointers for including exercise in your daily routine:

Start slowly: If you've never worked out before, start off cautiously and build up your workouts' duration and intensity gradually. This will help you maintain your health and prevent burnout.

Find activities you enjoy: Exercise doesn't have to be a much of a hard work. Find activities that you enjoy, like dancing, hiking, or playing sports, and incorporate them into your workout routine.

Set realistic goals: Set attainable objectives for yourself and monitor your development over time. This can help you stay motivated and make steady progress toward achieving your fitness goals.

Make it a habit: Try to incorporate exercise into your daily routine, whether that's by taking a walk during your lunch break or doing a quick workout before work. Making exercise a habit can help you stick to your South Beach Diet plan over the long term.

Get support: join a gym or fitness class, or find a workout buddy who can help keep you accountable and motivated. Having support can make a big difference when it comes to sticking to your fitness routine and achieving your goals.

In summary, exercise is an important component of the South Beach Diet plan. It can help you burn calories, build lean muscle mass, and increase metabolism, all of which are essential for achieving and maintaining a healthy weight. By incorporating cardiovascular exercise, strength training, and flexibility training into your workout routine, and following the tips for incorporating exercise into your lifestyle, you can support your South Beach Diet plan and achieve your fitness goals.

Remember, it's important to consult with your doctor before starting any new exercise program, especially if you have any health concerns or medical conditions. By combining a healthy diet with regular exercise, you can create a balanced and sustainable approach to weight loss and overall health and wellness.

CHAPTER 8

Frequently Asked Questions about the South Beach Diet

Q: What is the South Beach Diet, and how does it work?

A: Popular weight-loss plan The South Beach Diet is a low-carbohydrate, high-protein diet that emphasizes healthy fats, lean proteins, and complex carbohydrates. The diet is divided into three phases, with each phase gradually introducing different types of foods. The goal of the South Beach Diet is to promote weight loss, reduce inflammation, and improve overall health.

Q: Does the South Beach Diet work to help you lose weight?

A: Yes, the South Beach Diet can be an effective weight loss program. Studies have shown that the diet can lead to significant weight loss in both the short and long term. Like any weight reduction programme, though, specific results may vary.

Q: What are the key principles of the South Beach Diet?

A: The South Beach Diet is based on several key principles, including:

Emphasizing healthy fats, such as olive oil and nuts
Including lean proteins like fish and chicken
Limiting carbohydrates, especially those that are high in sugar and refined flour
Gradually reintroducing carbohydrates in later phases of the diet

Avoiding processed foods and sugary beverages
Encouraging regular exercise

Q: *What are the South Beach Diet's three stages?*
A: The South Beach Diet contains three phases, which are:

Phase 1: The strictest phase of the diet, which lasts for two weeks and eliminates most carbohydrates, including fruit, bread, pasta, and alcohol. During this phase, dieters focus on consuming lean proteins, healthy fats, and non-starchy vegetables.

Phase 2: This phase lasts until dieters reach their desired weight loss goal. During this phase, dieters gradually reintroduce carbohydrates back into their diet, including whole grains, fruits, and some starchy vegetables.

Phase 3: This is the maintenance phase of the diet, which is designed to be followed for life. During this phase, dieters continue to eat a healthy and balanced diet that emphasizes whole foods, lean proteins, healthy fats, and complex carbohydrates.

Are there any potential downsides to the South Beach Diet?

Like any diet, the South Beach Diet has its potential downsides. Some people may find it difficult to stick to the strict restrictions of Phase 1, and may experience side effects like headaches, fatigue, and constipation. Additionally, the diet can be more expensive than a typical diet, as it emphasizes high-quality proteins and healthy fats.

Q: Can the South Beach Diet be adapted for vegetarians or vegans?

A: Yes, the South Beach Diet can be adapted for vegetarians or vegans. In Phase 1, vegetarians can focus on consuming plant-based proteins like tofu, tempeh, and legumes, while vegans can focus on consuming a variety of plant-based proteins like tofu, tempeh, nuts, and seeds. In later phases of the diet, vegetarian and vegan dieters can gradually reintroduce complex carbohydrates like whole grains, fruits, and starchy vegetables.

Q: Is the South Beach Diet safe for people with diabetes or other health conditions?

A: The South Beach Diet can be a safe and effective weight loss program for people with diabetes or other health conditions. However, it's important to consult with a doctor before starting any new diet or exercise program, especially if you have any health concerns or medical conditions. Additionally, it's important to monitor blood sugar levels closely and make any necessary adjustments to medication or insulin doses.

In summary, the South Beach Diet is a popular and effective weight loss program that emphasizes healthy fats, lean proteins, and complex carbohydrates

CHAPTER 9

Tips for Long-term Success With The Diet

Focus on whole, nutrient-dense foods. The South Beach Diet encourages you to eat foods that are rich in nutrients, such as lean proteins, healthy fats, and complex carbohydrates. You'll feel content and full after eating these foods, which also give your body the nutrition it needs to function properly.

1. Meal plan and prep. Planning and prepping your meals in advance can help you stay on track with the South Beach Diet. Take some time each week to plan out your meals and snacks, and prep as much as you can in advance. This will help you avoid making

impulsive food choices when you're hungry and short on time.

2. Stay hydrated. Drinking a lot of water is very vital to your weight loss journey and not just that but your general health. Aim to drink at least 8-10 glasses of water per day, and consider adding in other low-calorie beverages like herbal tea and seltzer water.

3. Incorporate regular exercise. Exercise is an important component of the South Beach Diet, as it can help you burn calories, build lean muscle mass, and increase metabolism. Aim to incorporate both cardio and strength training into your fitness routine, and try to get at least 30 minutes of exercise most days of the week.

4. Practice mindful eating. Mindful eating involves paying attention to your body's hunger and fullness cues, and being present and focused while eating. You'll be able to eat less and choose your meals more carefully if you do this.

5. Stay accountable. Joining a support group or working with a dietitian can help you stay accountable and motivated on the South Beach Diet. Consider joining an online support group or working with a registered dietitian to help you achieve your weight loss and health goals.

By following these tips, you can set yourself up for long-term success with the South Beach Diet. Keep in mind that losing weight is a journey, so be persistent and patient with yourself. With time and dedication, you can achieve your weight loss and health goals on the South Beach Diet.

Conclusion

The South Beach Diet is a well-known and popular diet plan that has helped many people achieve their weight loss goals while also improving their overall health. By focusing on lean proteins, healthy fats, and complex carbohydrates, the South Beach Diet offers a balanced approach to eating that can lead to sustained weight loss and improved health.

While following the South Beach Diet, it's important to stay motivated and focused on your goals. Here are some tips to help you succeed on the South Beach Diet:

Plan ahead. By planning your meals in advance and having healthy snacks on hand, you can avoid making poor food choices when you're hungry and pressed for time.

Get assistance. When trying to follow a diet plan, having the support of family and friends can really help. Think about finding a partner to hold accountable or joining a group for support to help you remain inspired and on track.

Stay active. Exercise is an important part of any weight loss plan, and the South Beach Diet is no exception. Try to get at least 30 minutes of physical activity each day, whether it's walking, jogging, cycling, or another form of exercise that you enjoy.

Be patient. Losing weight takes time, and it's important to be patient and stay focused on your goals. Don't get discouraged if you don't see immediate results; stick with the plan and you will see progress over time.

Stay hydrated. Drinking plenty of water is essential for good health and can also help you feel full and satisfied. Aim for at least eight glasses of water a day, and try to limit your intake of sugary drinks and other high-calorie beverages.

By following these tips and staying committed to the South Beach Diet, you can achieve your weight loss goals and improve your overall health and wellbeing. Remember to be patient, stay motivated, and make healthy choices every day, and you will see the results you desire. Best of luck on your journey to a healthier, happier you!

Made in United States
North Haven, CT
30 August 2023